Pressing
RESET
for
Dynamic Hips

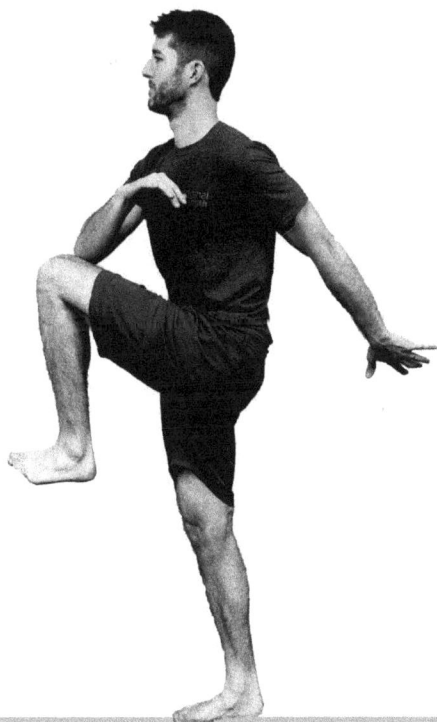

original
strength

original strength

Pressing RESET for Dynamic Hips

Published by OS Press - Fuquay-Varina, NC

Contributor:
Dan Bennett, PT, DPT, OCS, MTC, CMTPT, OS Certified Clinician

Photography by: Emily Lyons Selby, PT, DPT

ISBN: 979-8-9865860-7-6 (Paperback)

Thank you to JETLAUNCH.net for editing and book design.

Introduction

Having efficient hips is necessary for a healthy, dynamic life. We need our hips functioning well in order to walk, pick up our kids, care for our pets, run, and even throw a ball. Years of sitting in cars and at desks has done a disservice to our hip motion and strength. Most of us do not experience a variety of movements in our daily lives and regular activities. We begin to lose our natural birth right of dynamic movement.

Even if our hips don't hurt directly, the loss of movement at this critical joint can and will contribute to pain somewhere else in our body. This booklet is written for anybody looking to maintain or regain the function of their hips. You will be taught the principles of Original Strength and the Pressing RESET movement sequence. These techniques are wonderfully designed to allow for someone to get optimum function back to all the nooks and crannies of their hips. Whether you are a trainer, physical therapist, movement specialist, or someone who simply wants to move better, getting your hips working dynamically will restore motion you didn't even know you lost.

Medical Disclaimer: It is important to note that we are not here to diagnose or treat any medical or physical disorder. This is meant to be a guide to restoring healthy function to your hips and should not supersede any medical advice from your doctor or other health professionals that you work with. Do not move into pain. Pain is an alarm system telling your body that something is or may be wrong and needs to be respected. Our bodies compensate and move very differently when we are in pain. As we move more, and better, your body should improve but if you cannot perform the movements in this guide without pain then seek a medical professional.

Pressing
RESET

Our hips serve as vital connectors, link our trunk to the lower extremity. They play a pivotal role in facilitating a dynamic and active life of movement. The hips are a wonderfully designed joint that allow us a tremendous amount of mobility and strength. Our hips supply the power needed for moving forward while walking, sprinting uphill, sitting and standing from a chair, cutting while running, and gracefully spinning during a dance.

When our hips have the mobility and strength they are supposed to, they do a great job of generating and managing tremendous amounts of force. Force on the hip joint while walking can range from 1.8 to 3.8 times our body weight. The average adult in the United States (men and women averaged) is 185.3 lbs. This means that on average a person can transmit up to 518 lbs of force through each hip in every step they take! **This same average adult takes about 4,000 steps in a day accumulating 2,072,000 lbs of force through each hip every day!** That's an immense amount of force and stress, but no need to worry - we are designed to handle it.

Our big and powerful gluteus maximus muscles (e.g., butt muscles) propel us forward and upward depending on the task. But they can also help generate force up into our arms and across our body through a stable and reflexively strong spine and core. Think about throwing a ball. It goes a lot further when you drive off your foot, right? Throwing speed starts with leg strength and balance, not arm strength.

This begins to illustrate the huge impact that the hips have on our body. When things go wrong either from a lack of mobility or strength standpoint, the consequences can be felt in the far reaches of our body. There's evidence to support that if even one muscle stops doing its job at the hip, forces can exceed 4 times an individual's body weight leading to dysfunction of the joint. **That same average 185.3 lb person now has 740 lbs of force at their hip every step or 2,960,000 over the course of a day!**

A loss of internal rotation - essentially when the thigh spins in - leaves us unable to fully extend our hips. This means our leg cannot fully go back behind our trunk while walking, therefore our step is shortened in length, losing power and efficiency. It can even rob our glutes of their full strength. A lack of hip flexion, knee to chest, limits our ability to get into a deep squat to get on and off the floor. A lack of strength of the rotators of the hip can lead to caving in of the knees and a potential ACL tear or general increased wear and tear on the knee. A difference in hip rotation when comparing the two sides of the body has been linked to increased low back pain. If the hips don't rotate, then how do we change direction? The motion still must come from somewhere. Typically, this is when we start to overstress our low back or the knee, resulting in new or more pain and injuries.

Along with the spine, our hips have gotten the short end of the stick with our modern society's habit of sitting. Don't get me wrong, I enjoy a comfortable chair, but our bodies aren't meant to sit with hips and knees bent to 90-degree angles for 8-12 hours a day. We are meant to move. One of the amazing parts of the human body is its adaptability, your body will respond to whatever you do, good or bad. **The limited variety of movement we experience on a day-to-day basis decreases the amount of good information we give our brains about our body. This impacts our brain's ability to control our body and move through our environment with the ease which we were designed to do. Said in a different way - move it or lose it.**

That's enough with the doom and gloom, for there is hope. And that hope is movement. Our bodies are designed to move, and when we respect our design, our bodies tend to respond. A movement restoration program called Original Strength, allows and encourages us to respect that "original" design, hence the name. Original Strength is based on the neuro-developmental sequence, how our bodies and nervous system naturally develop starting from birth. Nobody told infant you how to breathe, how to hold your head up, how to roll, or crawl, or walk. You just did it. **When we are young the hip socket isn't even fully formed, it's an imperfect cone. It's only through rocking, crawling, and eventually walking that our natural play as infants and kids fully form the hip socket. You formed your hips as kids, you can regain them as an adult.** This program takes us back through that sequence and knocks the dust off the nervous system to allow you to regain healthy hips and a healthy life.

Pressing
RESET

Pressing RESET

Pressing RESET and your original strength are based on three pillars:

1. Breathing with your diaphragm, or breathing with your belly.
2. Activating the vestibular system, your balance and sensory integration system.
3. Engage in contralateral movement patterns (crawling, walking, marching) or midline crossing movements (reaching across the body or moving limbs on the opposite side of the body).

These pillars are preprogrammed into our nervous system when we are born. As we grow and explore the world as infants and children, we are constantly engaging in these three pillars, we never take a day off. By constantly engaging in these pillars, we not only become strong and resilient, we also continuously nourish our nervous system. It is crucial to continue to engage in these pillars to keep ourselves healthy and strong throughout our lifespan. So how exactly do we engage these pillars to regain our strength and restore our hips to their full potential? We Press RESET.

1. Diaphragmatic breathing
2. Eye/head control
3. Rolling

4. Rocking

5. Crawling/contralateral movements

All five of these motions/movements can play an integral role in restoring hip function. With hip function restored you'll improve the quality of your life and ability to express a dynamic movement portfolio throughout your lifespan.

The Hips are the Connectors

Let's get a little more into how Original Strength (OS) improves your hips. Some knowledge of hip anatomy and its relationship to the spine and lower extremity will help to illuminate that.

The hip is a deep ball and socket joint with a lot of motion. Your femur (thigh bone) forms the ball and fits in the socket formed by the bones of the pelvis. In between the pelvic bones (ilium) sits the wedge-shaped sacrum. These bones then form the sacroiliac joint and complete the ring-shaped pelvis which is the base for the spine, and as such your hips and spine are inextricably linked.

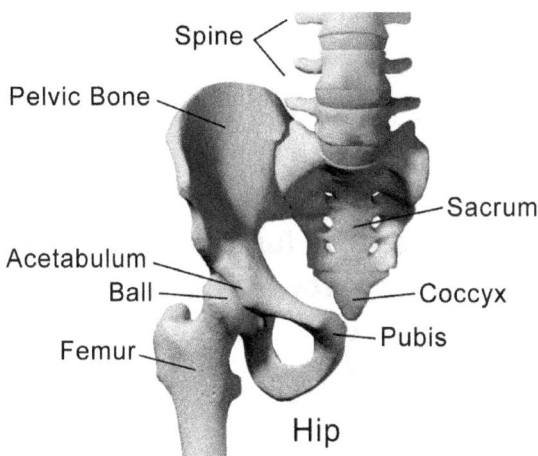

Hip

Your hip can flex (knee to chest), extend (kick behind you), rotate in and out, abduct (move away from the body) and, finally, adduct (move across the body). That's a substantial amount of motions requiring a lot of different muscles, and it comes with a big caveat. The socket of the hip sits at an oblique angle. What this means is that even when it looks like your hip is just moving one direction, like when moving your knee to your chest, it's actually moving around three different axes of motion. **This is a crucial point, in order to have full flexion of the hip, the hip must also rotate and glide to the side. We need to explore and restore all our natural motion in order to move optimally, not just live in a few basic straight line movements day in and day out.**

It is impossible to take your hip to its end range and not produce motion in the low back or pelvis which, again, emphasizes the importance of maximizing hip motion to minimize stress to other areas of the body.

We have 25 different muscles that have a direct attachment to the hip with the goal to either help move or stabilize the joint. Lack of activity offers a lot of opportunity for muscles to tighten up or get weaker, thereby reducing motion of the hip. **And remember, if even one hip muscle stops functioning it increases weight bearing forces through the hip!** We have cartilage in our hip joint which helps to manage these forces, dysfunction of the muscles therefore leads to early breakdown of this cartilage.

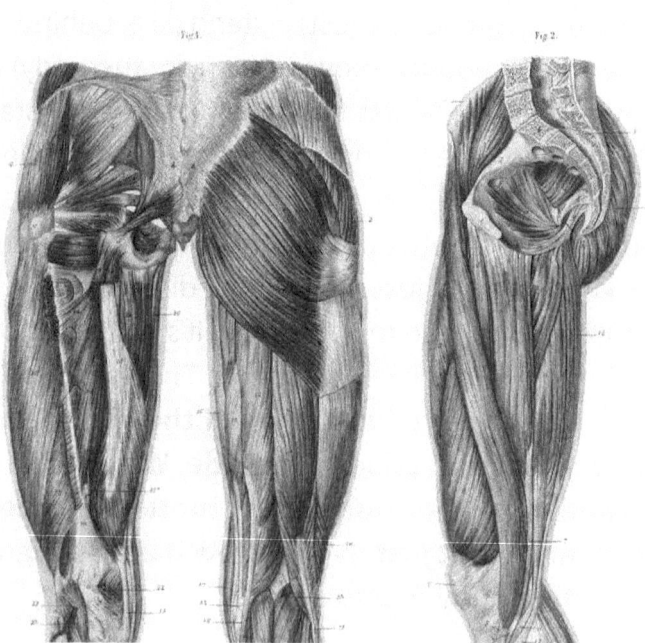

The hip also has an extensive capsule and ligament network to stabilize it. The hip is a ball and socket joint just like the shoulder, but unlike the shoulder which is likened to a golf ball sitting on a tee, the hip is a very deep and stable joint partially due to the capsule and ligament network. **The fiber orientation of the capsule develops while in the womb with the hips curled up tight to our body. This gives the hip ligaments a unique design with three different bands that form a spiral in standing. This contributes significantly to hip stability in standing and illustrates the beauty of our natural design that starts even before you were born.**

Adding to the dynamics of the joint capsule is the labrum. This is a ring of cartilage deepening the socket, however it does much more than improve stability. The labrum helps to provide pressurization and proprioceptive information regarding hip position and movement. **What that means is, the more we move, the more we stimulate the nerve endings, the better information we get from our hip about where we are in space which leads to better balance, movement and muscle function.** The more information we can give our brain, the better movement it helps produce.

Let's move on and highlight some of those muscles. Of particular importance is the psoas major muscle. The psoas major is a powerful hip flexor that runs from the front of the low back to the inside of the femur. What's unique and particularly important to OS, is that it has a direct tissue attachment to the diaphragm. So the better the diaphragm works, the better the psoas works and vice versa.

If either the diaphragm or psoas becomes dysfunctional it will affect the position of our femur altering all our weight bearing activities. When the psoas gets tight, we lose hip extension, glutes don't activate as well, and our low back and knees are under more stress and become overtaxed leading to injury. The psoas can get tight because it will try to assist the diaphragm with breathing. In order to optimize the psoas and the hip, the diaphragm must be functioning efficiently to prevent psoas tightness from recurring. Address the issue, not the symptom. Diaphragmatic breathing makes more sense now, right?

Speaking of glutes, we have three gluteal muscles and all are important. Our gluteus maximus is the star of the show and is what extends the hips and pushes us forward and upward. The fibers of the gluteus maximus are continuous with the ligaments of our sacroiliac joint (pelvis) and thus play a crucial role in stability of the pelvis and lumbar spine. Optimizing our glutes literally leads to a more stable pelvis and spine. Just as important though are our gluteus medius and minimus which sit on the side of the pelvis. These muscles help to stabilize our pelvis, hip and low back while working in concert with the quadratus lumborum muscle (QL) on the opposite side of the body forming a functional synergy - a group of muscles working together to create or prevent motion. Here we can begin to see the importance of both sides of the body communicating with each other. If the gluteus medius and gluteus minimus on the left side of the pelvis aren't carrying their load, that overtaxes the right side QL, and now we have a tightened, irritated muscle that just so happens to attach to our ribs, low back and shares a rib attachment with the diaphragm. This now impacts our breathing. Weakness here also leads to poor control of the femur causing the knee to cave in increasing the potential for knee injury.

Healthy hips are crucial to a healthy spine. If we begin to lose some of the motion that our hips are supposed to have, the low back often feels the brunt of that. As you sit, stand, twist, change direction, sprint or do basically any movement that requires hip motion and you don't have it, then over time, your back and knees pay the price. So, without further ado, let's get moving.

Pressing
RESET

Diaphragmatic Breathing

The diaphragm is a dome shaped muscle that sits underneath our rib cage. It has attachments to our lower ribs, lumbar spine, and even the ligament that surrounds the aorta (major blood vessel in the abdomen). The diaphragm also has important connections to our psoas major (hip muscle) and quadratus lumborum (low back muscle). Suffice to say, the diaphragm has some critical attachments and utilizing it as our primary breathing muscle, as we are designed to, is of great importance to our health. Not only is it designed to be our primary breathing muscle but it's also a key cog in our core, providing strength and stability to our spine, pelvis and hips.

Movement #1

HOOKLYING DIAPHRAGMATIC BREATHING

- If this is new to you, start on your back with your knees bent and in a relaxed position.

- Swallow and pay attention to where your tongue goes, it should raise to the roof of your mouth behind your top teeth. This is the natural resting position for your tongue and helps to facilitate breathing with your diaphragm and stabilizing muscles of the neck.

- Rest your hands on your stomach to help detect the movement of air.

- Breathe in through your nose, direct the flow of air into your stomach and feel your stomach and lower rib cage expand.

- The muscles in your neck and upper chest should be relaxed.

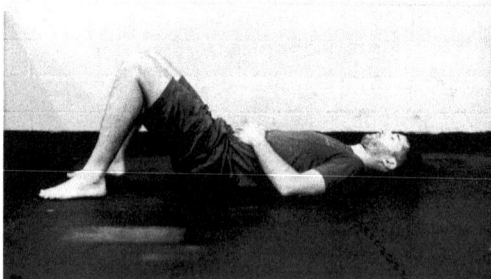

Once you get the hang of movement #1, there are two alternate positions that can help with two commonly restricted hip positions.

Movement #2

HAPPY BABY BREATHING

Many of us are missing our full range of hip flexion (knees to chest) despite all the sitting we do and this impacts our ability to squat. This position shortens the diaphragm and pushes your abdominal contents up into the diaphragm promoting a mild stretch that can be faciliatory to the diaphragm. This can make it easier for some people to breathe into the belly.

- Lay on your back and bring both knees as far towards your chest as possible.
- Breathe in through your nose, direct the flow of air into your stomach and feel your stomach and lower rib cage expand.
- The muscles in your neck and upper chest should be relaxed.

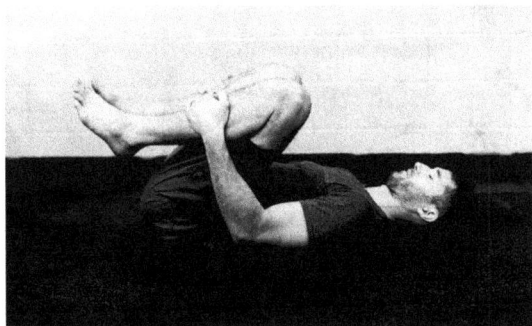

Movement #3

PRONE DIAPHRAGMATIC BREATHING/ALLIGATOR BREATHING

- Another great position is laying on your belly with your forehead resting on your wrists.

- Breathe in through your nose, direct the flow of air into your stomach and feel your stomach and lower rib cage expand.

- The muscles in your neck and upper back and chest should be relaxed.

This position promotes hip extension which is lost in a lot of us with the amount of desk work and driving we do. The other advantage of this position is that it provides increased sensation as we can feel our body weight pushing our belly into the floor as we breathe, increasing our awareness and enhancing diaphragmatic function.

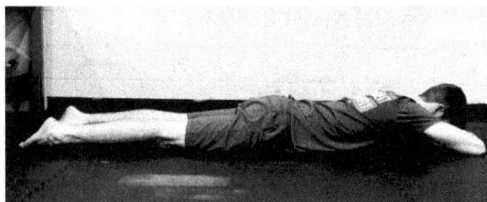

Whatever position you choose, pick the one that feels the easiest to promote pure belly breathing with a relaxed neck. Perform for 2 minutes. Don't make every breath a deep breath, no need to hyperventilate. Throw a few deep breaths in there but try to make your normal, everyday breath come from the belly.

Eye and Head Control

Movement of the head and neck are great for stimulating our vestibular system and mobilizing the spine. By moving the eyes and head we provide a plethora of information to our brain about where we are in space and this, in turn, helps our balance. **The more active our vestibular system, the more efficiently our brain communicates with all of our muscles, especially those of the core, hips and ankles which are constantly active to help keep us upright and from falling over.** The more mobile the spine is, the better our hips can interact with it.

Here's how:

Movement #1

PRONE ON ELBOWS HEAD ROTATIONS AND NODS

- Lay prone, on your belly, propped up onto your elbows and rotate your head as far as you can comfortably to the left, and then back to the right.

- Lead the motion with your eyes, look to the left first then rotate your head.

- Make sure your tongue stays on the roof of your mouth and you maintain diaphragmatic breathing.

- After 10 reps side to side switch to looking up and down.

- Only look up as far as you can comfortably and without pain in the neck.

- This position helps get our hips into extension which is very often lost due to sitting.

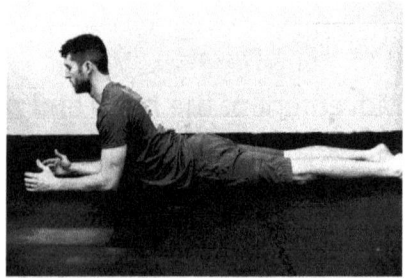

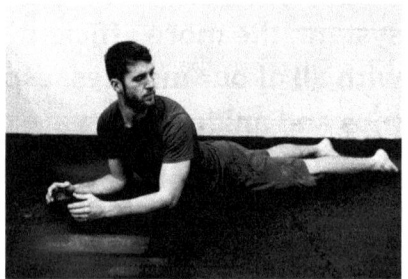

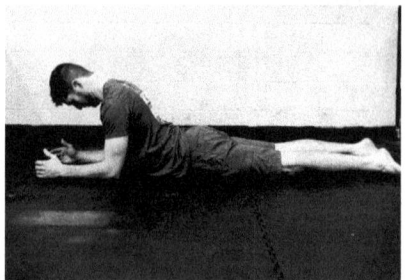

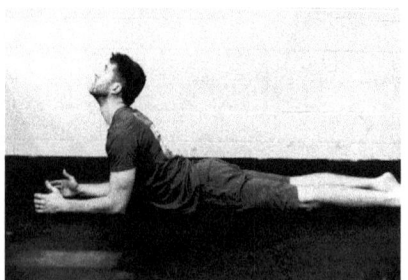

Movement #2

ROCKED BACK HEAD ROTATIONS AND NODS

- An alternate position is quadruped with hips rocked back.

- Perform the same motions of looking up and down. You can feel the muscles further down in your back contract as you look up and your lats contract as you rotate side to side

- This position helps get the hips into a deeper/higher degree of flexion which is often missing leading to stress on the low back and difficulty with squatting and getting in/out of your car.

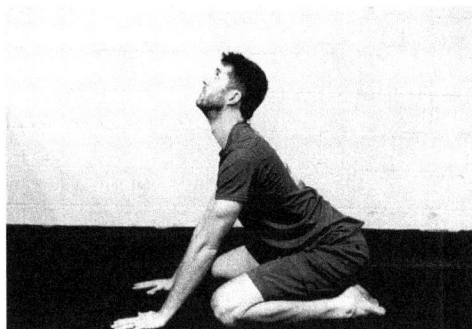

RESET #3

Rolling

Rolling is a massively important part of our developmental process, it's a foundational movement. We all rolled before we ever crawled or walked. Rolling lays the neurological foundation for walking, connects our shoulders to the core to the opposite hip, and prepares us for rotational tasks like throwing, sprinting, getting on and off the floor, or swinging a golf club. Rolling ties the body together leading to rotational strength and stability.

Rolling creates rotation in the spine which it needs for nourishment to stay healthy and vibrant throughout our lifespan. The rotation appropriately tenses the discs in your spine which helps to strengthen them thereby keeping them healthy.

It stimulates the vestibular and proprioceptive systems, giving your brain an abundance of information about where your body is in space and deepens your head control. This in turn helps to improve balance, sensation, and coordination which helps with all tasks. Rolling is going to help facilitate and mobilize your hips in ways other movements just can't do. This new range of motion and motor control will make your hips dynamic once again.

Let's roll:

Movement 1

EGG ROLLS WITH GROIN MUSCLE EMPHASIS

- Lay on your back with knees pulled up to your chest.

- Mouth closed, tongue on the roof of your mouth.

- Look to the side, then rotate your head to the same side, then let the rest of your body roll with you.

- Continue to rotate the head and neck as far as you can comfortably once on your side to get as much rotation as possible.

- Rotate your head the opposite direction and pull your legs with you creating a roll.

- As you rotate to the opposite you can get a little extra stretch to the groin muscles by allowing the legs to separate and utilizing the pull on the groin muscles to assist your body rolling back over along with the head.

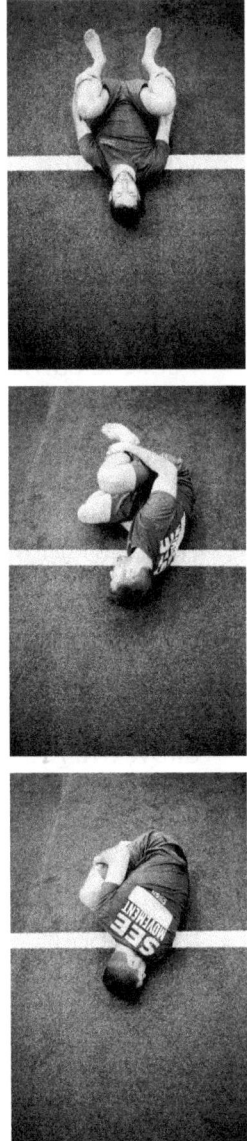

Movement #2

FULL UE SEGMENTAL ROLL

- Lay on your back with one hand raised in front of your shoulder.

- Mouth closed, tongue on the roof of your mouth.

- Reach across your body and drive your head across your body to promote the roll onto your stomach.

- Feel the same side glute muscle engage and you promote the reciprocal action required for gait.

- Keep your eyes on your hand as you roll onto your stomach.

- From your stomach reach behind your head.

- Keep your eyes on your hand and allow the movement of your head and shoulder girdle to roll you back onto your back.

- Maintain diaphragmatic breathing throughout.

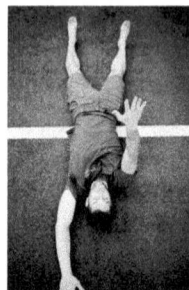
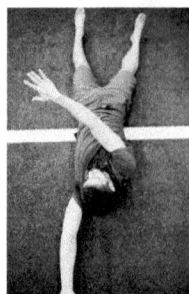
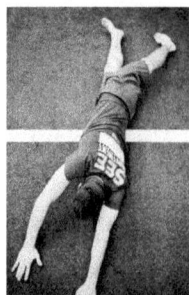
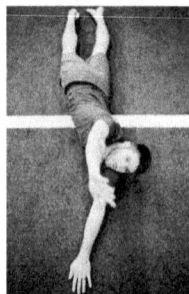

Movement #3

FULL LE SEGMENTAL ROLL

- Laying on your back bring your knee towards your chest making your hip a 90-degree angle.

- Tongue on the roof of your mouth, breathing through your nose.

- Kick your leg across your body promoting a roll onto your belly.

- From your stomach bend your knee and lift the thigh off the ground, thinking about reaching across your body with your foot.

- Allow your spine to rotate and your leg to take you back onto your back.

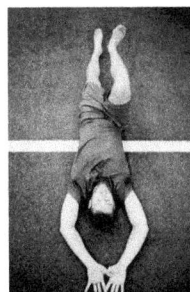

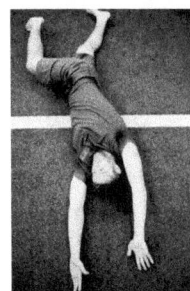

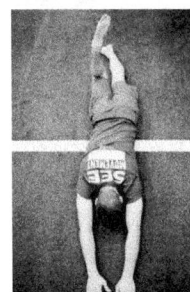

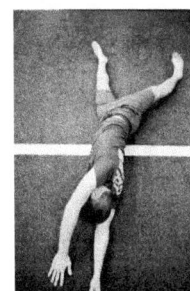

Movement #4

LE PRONE HALF ROLL

- We can really emphasize glute activation by doing just half a roll from our belly.

- Start by lying flat on your stomach.

- Tongue on the roof of your mouth, breathing through your nose.

- Bend your knee and lift your thigh off the ground reaching across your body, allowing the spine to rotate and then return to the starting position.

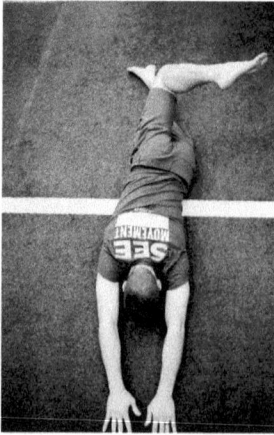

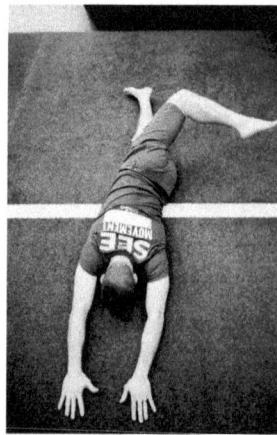

Movement #5

ELEVATED ROLL

- This roll increases the intensity and can promote strengthening to the side of the hips to assist with stability of the pelvis and low back with walking.

- Start in a push up position.

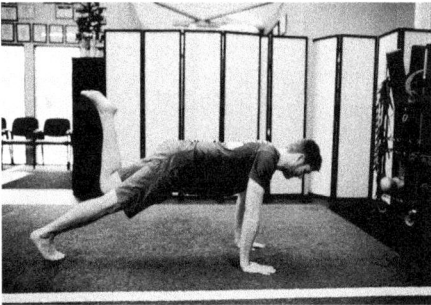

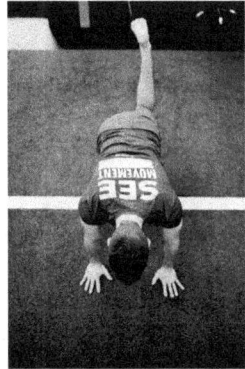

- Tongue on the roof of your mouth, breathing through your nose.

- Bend one knee and reach across your body until the toe touches the ground.

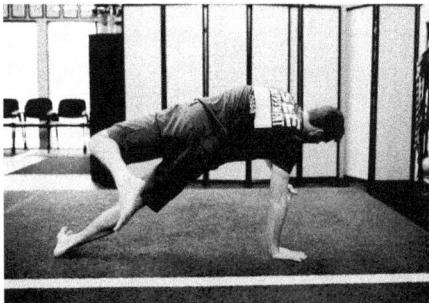

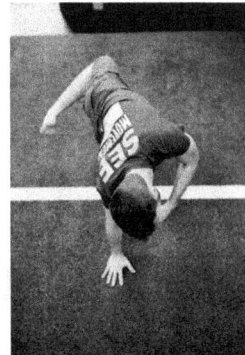

- Reach with the same side arm up towards the ceiling, keep your eyes on your hand.

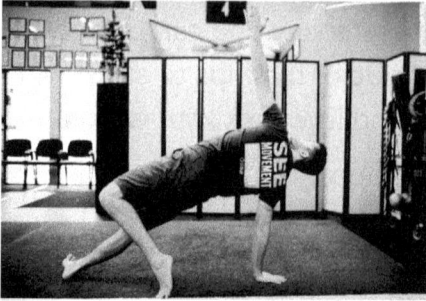

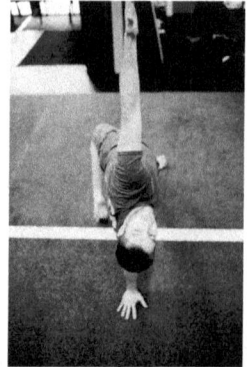

- Feel the strength and hold strong with the down shoulder and hip.

For a fun variation do it from your forearms. This engages the serratus anterior muscle, which blends with the obliques, which blends with core and hip muscles on the opposite side of the body promoting entire body work. Human body connectivity at its finest. Think of scooping your forearm along the ground towards your body to really feel the muscles on the side of the shoulder and trunk engage.

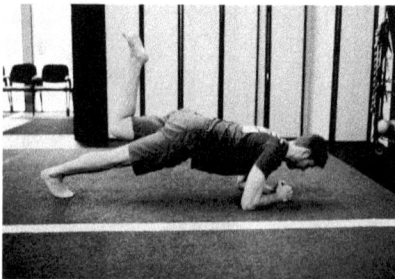

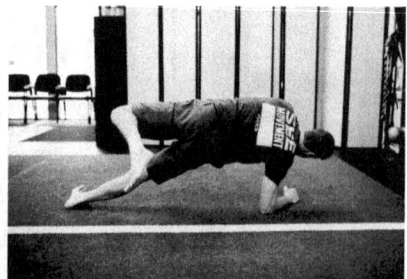

Pressing RESET for Dynamic Hips

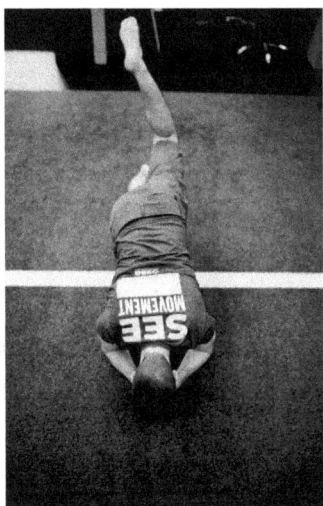

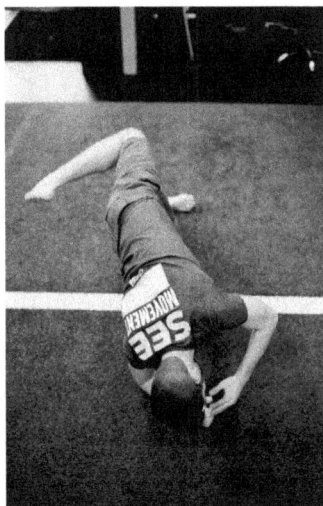

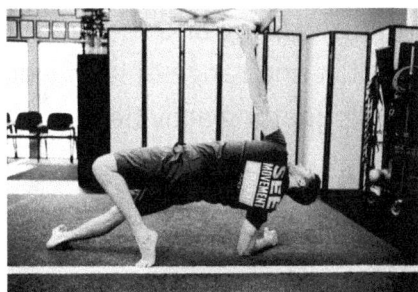

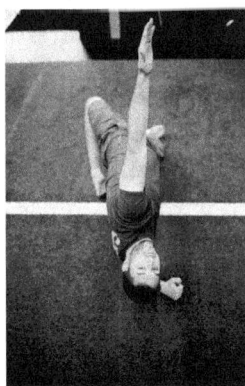

RESET #4

Rocking

Rocking on our hands and knees is some of the first weight bearing we do as infants, and it promotes stability of both the shoulder and hip girdles. Weight bearing through our extremities causes joint compression, which nourishes the joints, and automatically fires the stabilizing muscles of the joints. **As mentioned earlier, when we are first born our hip socket isn't fully formed, it is through weight bearing that the head of the femur helps to form the socket. Rocking returns us to the movements that literally formed the hip socket.**

Rocking promotes the transfer of force from legs to shoulders and vice versa, through a stable core. This helps to train our core to do what it's designed to do, stabilize the spine and conduct force from one limb to another which prepares us for crawling, walking and running. This reset also helps develop the lost end range of hip flexion which is required for efficient squatting activities.

Movement #1

QUADRUPED ROCKING

- Start on your hands and knees.

- Tongue on the roof of your mouth, breathing through your nose.

- Start with toes pointed away from you.

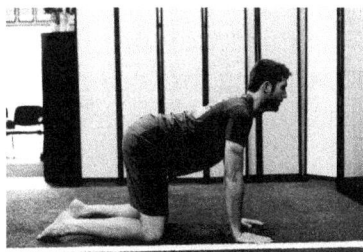

- Rock forward keeping your elbows straight and a tall proud sternum, you should feel some muscle activity in the shoulders and core.

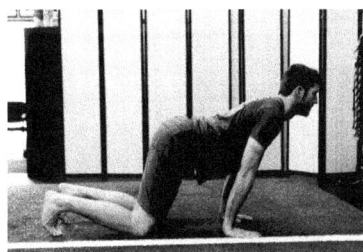

- Keep the head up as much as comfortable, don't crane to look at the ceiling but don't look at the floor either.

- Rock your hips back to your ankles, maintain the natural curve in your spine, don't round into a prayer stretch. This ensures the hips go into flexion and enhances our

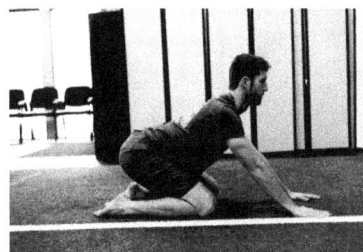

ability to squat. If your back starts to round you've stopped stretching your hips and are now just bending the spine, which is not what we are looking for here.

- Perform again with toes curled underneath you to get a different stretch into the ankles.

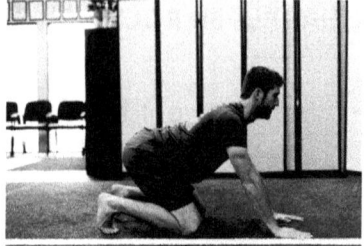

- Lateral variation: In this same position instead of shifting forward and back, shift side to side to get other corners of your hip.

- Circle variation: In this same position make circles to get much needed rotation back to your hips.

Movement #2

ROCKING WITH HIPS IN ROTATION

- Starting in the same quadruped position, swing both feet out to the left, perform 10 reps then swing your feet to the right.

- As before, rock back and forth as far as you can comfortably, do not go into pain, you will feel stretching in your hips, this new position helps to restore rotation to the hip.

  » Medical disclaimer: If you have recently had your hip replaced do not perform this variation.

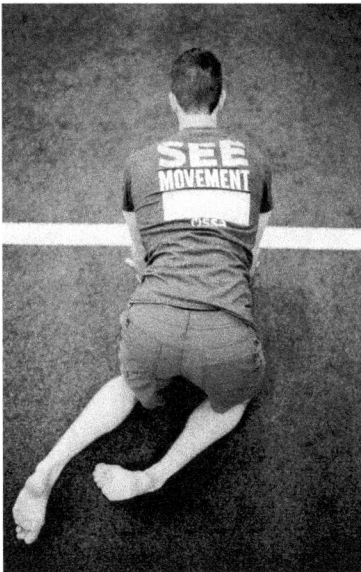

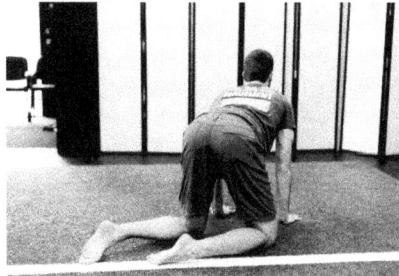

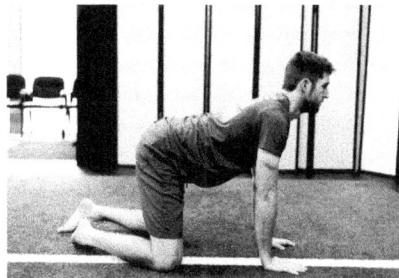

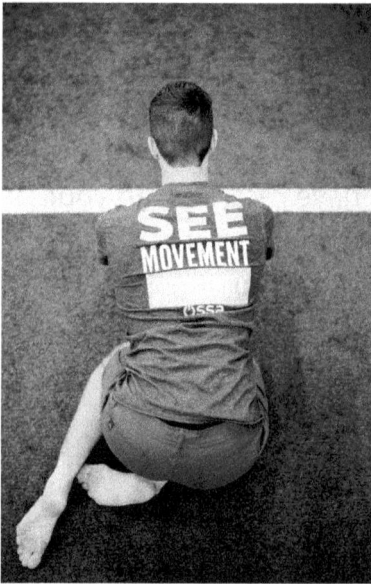

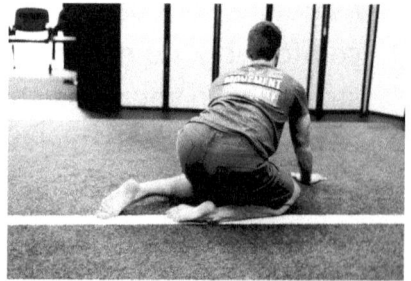

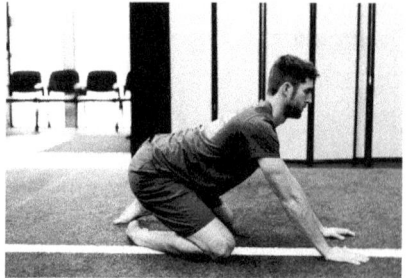

Pressing RESET for Dynamic Hips

Movement #3

LEGO ROCKING

- This is a great position to really challenge and improve hip mobility more than rocking on hands and knees.

- Get in the position pictured.

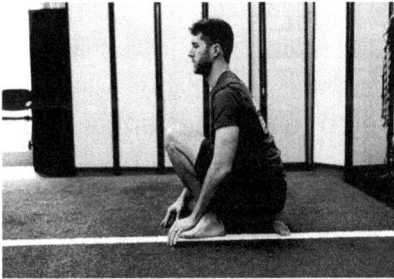

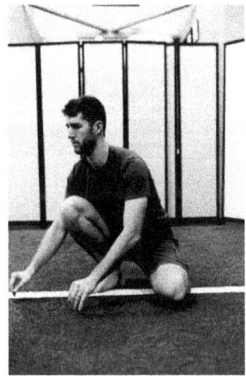

- Tongue on the roof of your mouth, breathing through your nose.

- Shift your body forward into the top leg as if to initiate crawling.

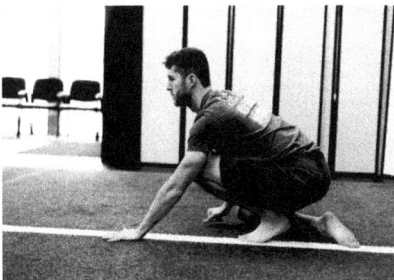

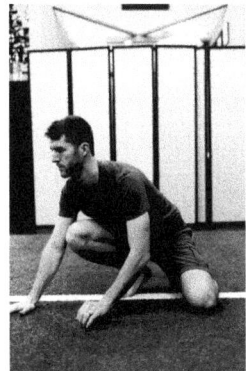

- This forces the top knee down to the floor, shifting weight to and stretching the foot.

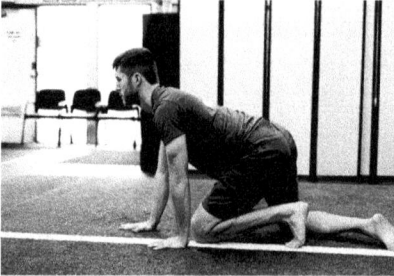

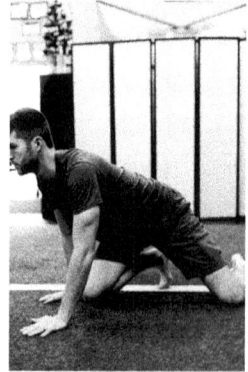

- You can change the stretch to the foot/ankle and hip by having the knee either inside or outside the elbow. Do whatever feels good!

RESET #5

Crawling

Crawling is where everything gets tied together. It builds upon the foundation laid with rocking. In rocking, we were connecting the shoulders and hips through the core, but now we really build some forward momentum. Crawling promotes contralateral limb activity necessary for walking, running, throwing and just about any dynamic task we perform. Force is generated with the opposite side arm and hip, transferred through our automatically and reflexively stable core to propel us forward. Coordinating effort between our hips and the opposite shoulder is a crucial developmental step. Crawling optimizes human movement. This progresses us perfectly into an upright gait where walking should be a four limbed activity coordinating the opposite arm and leg.

Movement #1

HANDS AND KNEES CRAWLING

- Begin in the same position as rocking, hands under shoulders, knees under hips.

- Reach forward with one arm and the opposite knee.

- Maintain diaphragmatic breathing, through the nose, with tongue on the roof of the mouth.

- Continue crawling for 2 minutes to build some endurance.

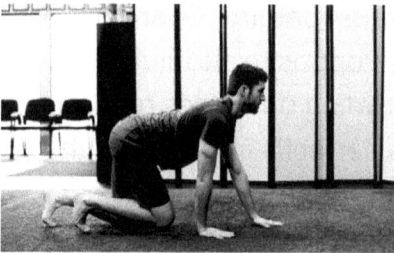

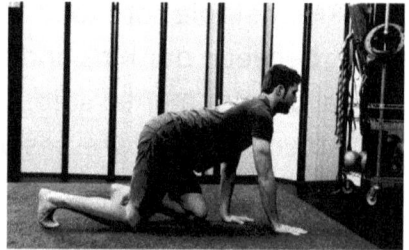

- Keep your head up.

- To add some intensity - leopard crawl. It's the same movement as hands and knees crawling but keep your knees in the air, butt below your shoulders.

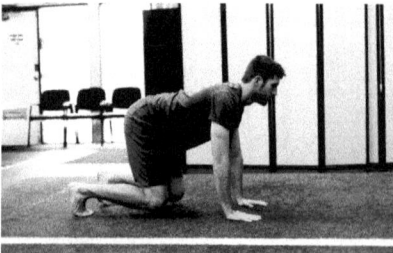

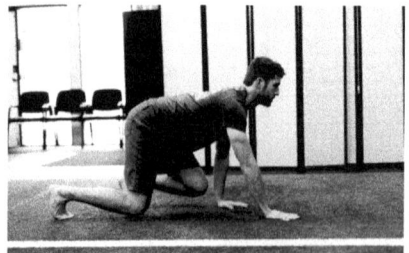

Movement #2

INFINITY CRAWLING

- Place two cones about 5 feet apart.

- Crawling in the same manner as before, weave in and out of the cones in the shape of the infinity symbol/ figure 8.

- This crawl promotes a lot of great weight bearing hip rotation that straight line crawling doesn't.

- Once again maintain breathing with your diaphragm.

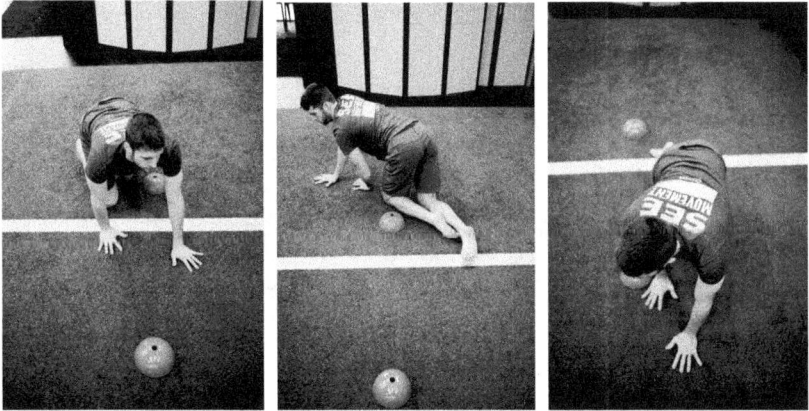

Movement #3

SPEED SKATERS

- Speed skaters are great at getting our hips into full extension which hands and knees crawling misses and more closely resembles our gait cycle.

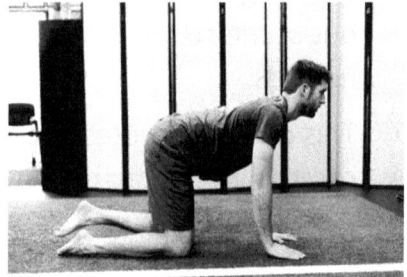

- Assume the quadruped position.

- Extend one hip and the opposite side shoulder.

- Return to the starting position and repeat with the opposite limbs.

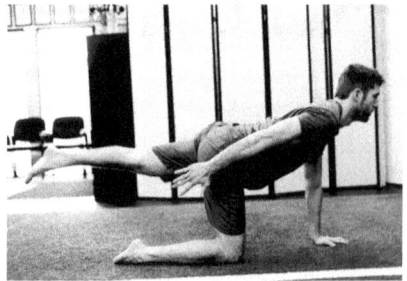

- Maintain diaphragmatic breathing and keep your head up.

Movement #4

STANDING CROSS CRAWL

- Standing with feet shoulder width apart, tongue on the roof of your mouth, breathing through your nose.

- Bring your opposite elbow and knee together in front of your body.

- Stand tall on the down leg, don't bring your trunk down to your knee, bring your knee up to you.

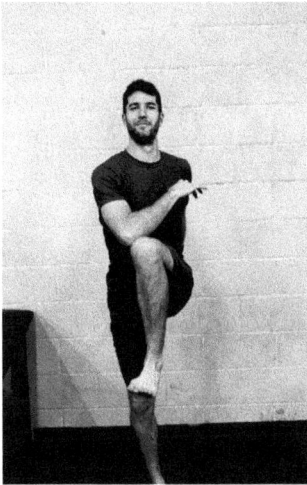

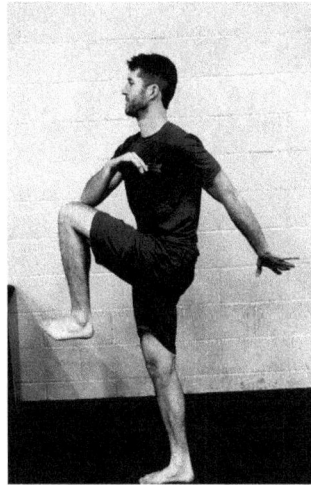

- If your elbow doesn't reach then use your forearm or hand.

- It's more important to stay upright to help engage your glutes on the leg you are standing on.

- Alternate back and forth.

Your
DESIGN

Daily Routine RESETS

10-minute Routine:

Prone diaphragmatic breathing, happy baby breathing to get hips to end ranges: 1' each
Prone on elbows (POE) with head rotations and nods, 10x each
Segmental rolling 3x each extremity
Happy baby roll 3x
Rocking with ankles pointed towards you 10x
Rocking with feet swung to the left and then right 10x each
Infinity crawling 2 minutes
Slow cross crawls 20x

15-minute routine:

Prone diaphragmatic breathing, happy baby breathing to get hips to end ranges: 1 minute each
Prone on elbows (POE) with head rotations and nods, 10x each
Supine UE half roll, 5x
Prone LE half roll, 5x
Segmental rolling 4x each extremity
Happy baby roll 3x
Rocking with ankles pointed towards you 10x
Rocking with feet swung to the left and then right, 10x each
Lego Rocking 5x each leg
Infinity crawling 2 minutes
Skaters 20x each side
Slow cross crawls 20x

If you want some intensity, add 1 minute of leopard crawl to either routine. It's one of the biggest bang for your buck exercises out there.

The Power in Your Design

Our bodies are beautifully designed to move throughout the world. We are meant to run, jump, climb, lift, spin and throw. **The position our hips are in while in utero creates a perfect twist in the ligaments to make us stable in standing. The original design is there, all we have to do is honor it.**

Unfortunately, the modern world we live in now doesn't ask us to use our bodies as they were designed. So, we have adapted to the demands of modern society. Luckily for us, **adaptation can go both ways**. If we challenge ourselves physically and honor our body, it will respond with strength and resilience. If we only put forth what is required from desk jobs and driving cars, we will adapt with tightness and weakness accordingly. Our hips take a huge toll from prolonged sitting day in, day out, and the effects of that can be wide ranging. Dysfunctional hips impact our ability to walk, squat, pick up our kids, run and even breath. By just taking a few minutes out of your day to perform purposeful movement you can flip the script, readapt and regain your Original Strength.

Want to learn more?

This booklet was designed to give a brief overview of the Original Strength System and how it can help you Press RESET on how you move to help your hips serve you for your lifetime.

We put it together because we know it can help everyone and anyone. If you do nothing more than what is in this booklet, you will notice many changes in how your mind and body begin to feel and react to various situations.

Original Strength is a human movement education company with a mission to bring the hope and strength of movement to every body in the world. Based on the human developmental sequence and the human body's design, the Original Strength System teaches movements that help RESET an individual's neuromuscular system, allowing them to enjoy improved physical movement and physiological function.

We conduct courses, training, and certify coaches and instructors. We also develop educational materials for PE teachers, physical therapy students, medical professionals, trainers, coaches fitness/health/wellness instructors, sports conditioning professionals, and individuals/groups working with vestibular and neuromuscular functionality.

If you want to know more about Pressing RESET and regaining your original strength, visit https://

originalstrength.net. There you will find a variety of books, hundreds of free video tutorials (**OS Movement Snax**), and a complete listing of our courses and OS Certified Professionals near you.

You may want to consider finding an OS Certified Professional. These professionals will conduct an Original Strength Screen and Assessment (OSSA), which is the quickest and easiest way to identify areas your movement system needs to go from good to best. The OSSA allows a pro to pinpoint the best place for you to start Pressing RESET and restoring your Original Strength.

We encourage you to reach out to the OS team with any questions you may have. ***Please keep us updated with your progress; we really want to know how you are doing - progress@OriginalStrength.net.***

Press RESET now and live life better & stonger because you were awesomely and wonderfully made to accomplish amazing things.

For more information:

original
strength

Original Strength Systems, LLC
OriginalStrength.net

PressingRESETfor@Originalstrength.net

original
strength

originalstrength.net

Published by

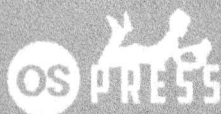
OS PRESS